CONTENTS

1: KETO CHICKEN AND WAFFLE SANDWICHES	1
2: LOW CARB ALMOND FLOUR WAFFLES	4
3: COCONUT CRUNCH WAFFLES	6
4: SWEET AND SAVOURY WAFFLE'S	8
5: CREAMY CHEESE KETO WAFFLES?	10
6: NEXT LEVEL SWEET AND SPICY CHAFFLES?	13
7: BEST KETO CHAFFLES	15
8: CRISPY, CHEESEY AND SPICY CHAFFLES WITH A TOUCH OF SWEETNESS IN IT..	17
9: DELICIOUS KETO CHAFFLES..	19
10: BLUE BERRIES CHAFFLE..	21
11: STANDARD CHAFFLE	23
12: CHOCOLATE CHIP COOKIE CHAFFLES..	26
13: BBQ KETO CHAFFLES	28
14: KETO CHICKEN BACON RANCH CHAFFLES..	30
15: EASY KETO CHAFFEL RECIPE..	32
16: KETO PIZZA STYLE CHAFFEL..	34
17: BROCCOLI AND CHEDDAR LOW CARB KETO WAFFLES..	37
18: LOW CARB KETO WAFFLES..	39
19: CAULIFLOWER WAFFLES..	41
20: SWEET POTATO WAFFLE'S..	44
21: PUMPKIN SPICE KETO CHAFFLES..	46
22: BACON, MUSHROOMS SMOKED CHAFFLES..	49
23: PECAN CINNAMON CHAFFEL WITH DELICIOUS CREAM CHEESE SOFTENING..	52
24: CHAFFEL PICKLE SPEARS..	55
25: VEGETABLE CHEESE CHAFFLE..	62
26: KETO GRILLED PEPPERONI CHAFFEL..	65
27: KETO FRENCH TOAST LIKE CHAFFLES...	68
28: CHOCOLATE PECAN CHAFFLE..	71
29: ORANGE CINNAMON ROLL CHAFFLE..	73
30: KETO CORN BREAD CHAFFLE..	76

Copyright © Stephanie Baker

All rights reserved. No part of this book may be reproduced, scanned or distributed in any printed or electronic form without permission. Please do not participate in or encourage piracy of copyrighted materials in violation of the author's rights. Purchase only authorized editions.

1: KETO CHICKEN AND WAFFLE SANDWICHES

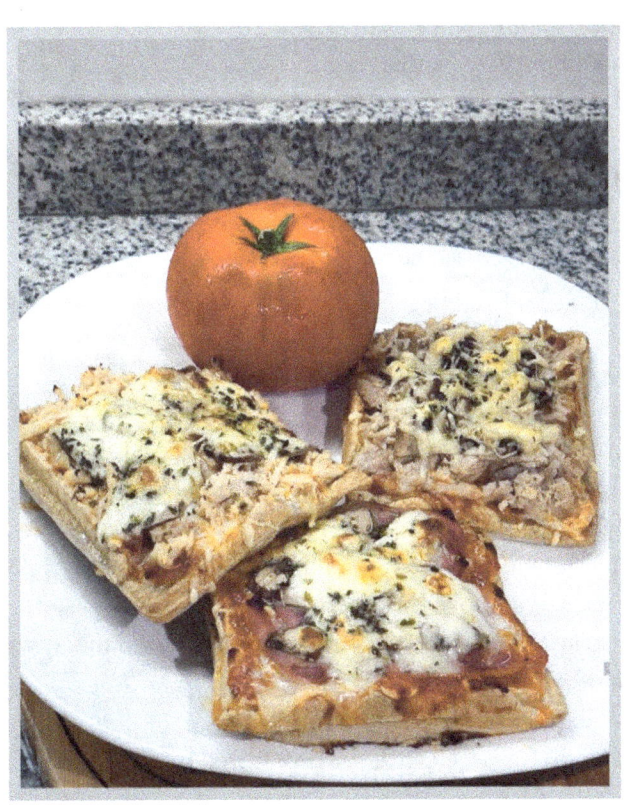

Ingredients

- 2 Chicken slices
- 1 Cup of Butter Milk
- Salt and black pepper ½ teaspoon
- ¼ teaspoon Cayenne
- 1 Large Egg
- 1 Cup of Almond Flour
- 2 tablespoons of Olive Oil

Waffle ingredients

- 3 Large size Eggs
- ¼ cup of milk
- 2 tablespoons of melted butter
- 1 tablespoon of vanilla essence
- 1 cup of almond flour, 1 teaspoon of Salt
- 2 Large eggs white
- Mustard paste 2 tablespoons
- Crispy Bacon's 3 teaspoons
- Cucumbers pickle slices ⅚
- Maple syrup 1 tablespoon

How to make keto and Waffle sandwiches???

1. Take two boneless chicken slices cut it into stripes
2. Put it in a dish and pour 1 cup of butter milk, soak it overnight
3. Remove chicken from the butter milk and then sprinkle some salt and black pepper
4. Also sprinkle some cayenne powder on it and mix it with your hands
5. Let it marinate for 5 minutes
6. Now take a large egg and whisk it well in a bowl

7. Take 1 cup of Almond flour, sprinkle some black pepper powder on it
8. Coat each piece of chicken with egg and almond flour
9. Repeat for two layers of breading
10. Take a pan and add some oil, cook chicken strips until golden
11. After frying bake them at 350F
12. Now get ready to make your waffles
13. Take 3 large size eggs and ¼ cup of milk
14. Take 2 tablespoons of melted butter, and 1 tablespoon of vanilla essence add them in egg mixture
15. Mix them well
16. Now take 1 cup of almond flour, 1 teaspoon of salt whisk it well until no lumps remains
17. Take 2 large eggs white, beat to stiff peaks
18. Carefully fold egg whites into waffle batter
19. Greece waffle iron
20. Pour the Waffle batter
21. Cook for 5-6 minutes until golden
22. Apply some mustard paste on the Waffle and put chicken pieces
23. Sprinkle crispy bacon and put slices of cucumber pickle, pour maple syrup

2: LOW CARB ALMOND FLOUR WAFFLES

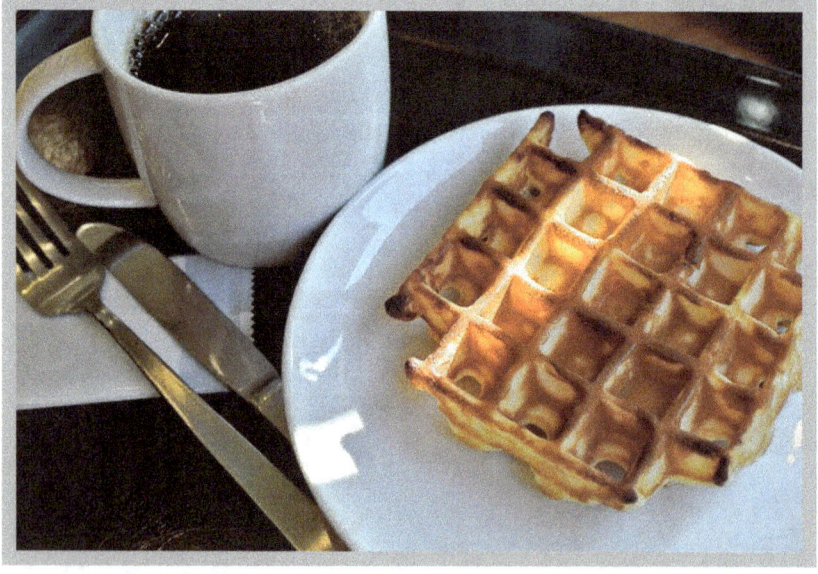

Ingredients

- 2 large eggs
- 2 tablespoons melted butter

- 1 tablespoon sweet almond milk
- ½ teaspoon of vanilla extract
- 4 tablespoons of super-fine natural almond flour
- 2 tablespoons of sugar (The ultimate sugar replacement)
- ½ teaspoon of baking powder and just a pinch of salt
- Low carbs pancake syrup 2 tablespoons HOW TO MAKE LOW CARB ALMOND FLOUR WAFFLES?
- Take a blender, add 5 eggs
- Pour a cup of melted butter
- Add 1 tablespoon of sweet almond milk
- Then add half teaspoon of vanilla extract
- Add 4 tablespoons of super-fine natural almond flour
- Add 2 tablespoons of sugar (the ultimate sugar replacement)
- Add ½ teaspoon of baking powder and a pinch of salt
- Blend these ingredients until thick batter forms
- Take a waffle maker spray some oil
- Pour chaffle batter cook them and pour o carb pancake syrup on it

3: COCONUT CRUNCH WAFFLES

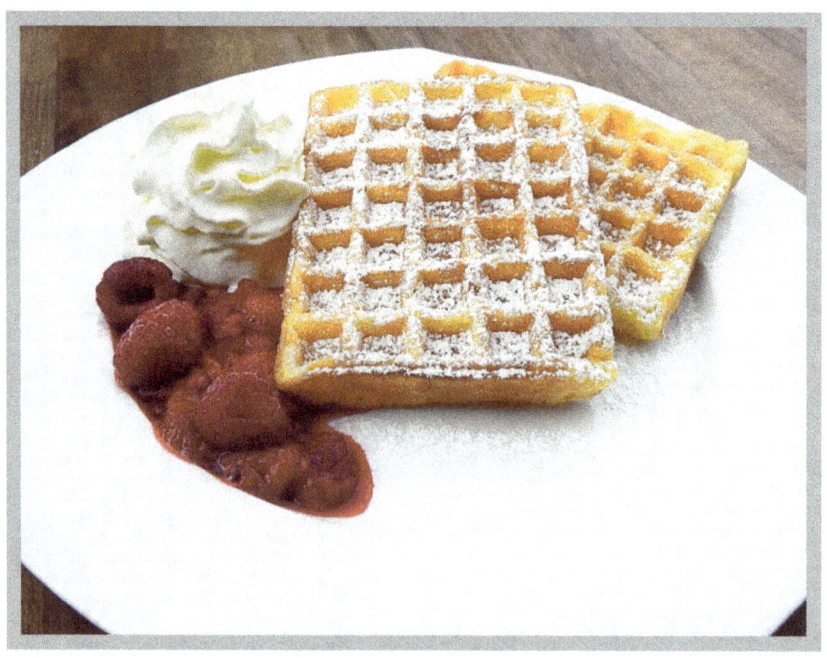

INGREDIENTS

1. 5 eggs
2. 1 Cup of melted butter
3. Half teaspoon of baking powder
4. Half teaspoon of salt
5. ⅛ teaspoon of sweet leaf Stevia drops or 2 packets of sweetener
6. ⅓ cup of coconut flour
7. Maple syrup 2 tablespoon
8. Almond crumbs 1 teaspoon

HOW TO MAKE COCONUT CRUNCH WAFFLES?

- Take a blender, add 5 eggs
- Pour a cup of melted butter
- Blend it up till it gets mixed
- Add half teaspoon of baking powder in it
- Add half teaspoon of salt
- Add ⅛ teaspoon of sweet leaf stevia drops / two packets sweetener
- Add ⅓ cup of coconut flour
- Add almond crumbs
- Blend it until it gets smooth and remain no lumps
- Take waffles maker spray with coconut oil
- Pour batter in it and cook it for 5-6 minutes
- After removing from waffle maker pour maple syrup on it

4:SWEET AND SAVOURY WAFFLE'S

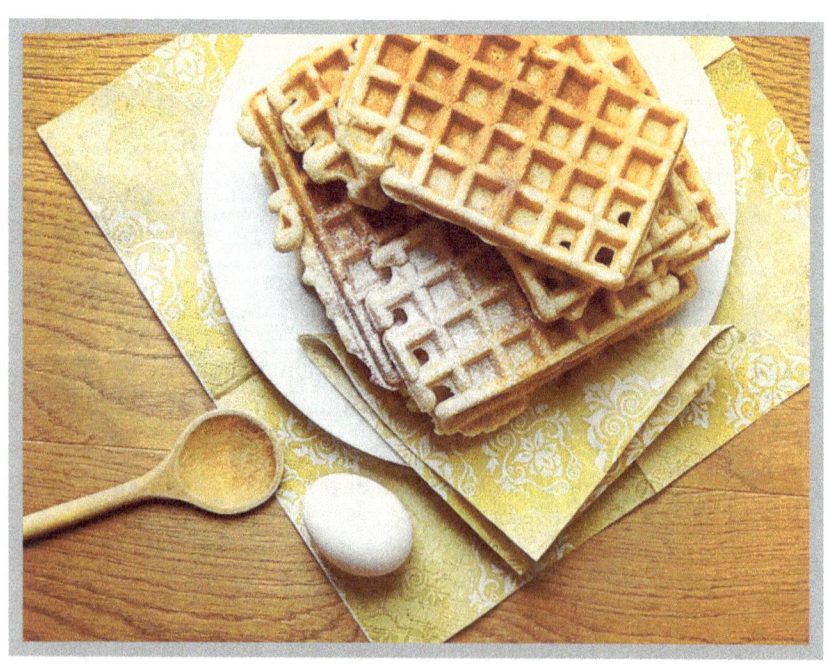

Ingredients

- 3 eggs
- ¼ cup of fiber yum
- Pinch of cayenne powder
- 1 teaspoon of honey
- 2 teaspoons of melted butter
- 3 tablespoons of multi grain oats powder
- ¼ teaspoon of garlic powder
- Maple syrup and sour cream

HOW TO MAKE SWEET AND SAVOURY WAFFLES?

- Take a blender, add eggs in it
- Add ¼ cup of fiber yum
- Add a pinch of cayenne powder
- Add 1 teaspoon of honey
- Add 2 teaspoons of melted butter
- Then add 3 tablespoons of multi grain oats powder
- Add ¼ teaspoons of garlic powder
- Blend it until no lumps remain
- Take a waffle maker and heat it up
- Spray some Avocado oil
- Pour chaffle batter on it and cook it for 5-6 minutes
- Remove from the iron and pour maple syrup

5: CREAMY CHEESE KETO WAFFLES?

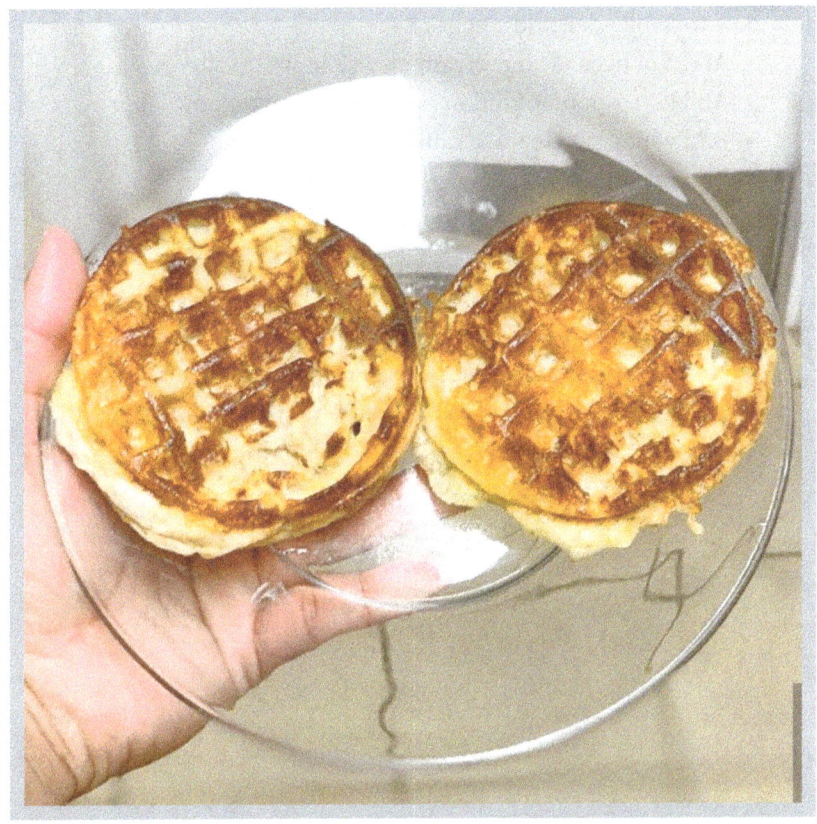

INGREDIENTS.

- 2 eggs
- 2 ounces sour cream cheese
- ½ teaspoon onion powder
- ½ teaspoon cinnamon powder
- Whipping cream ½ teaspoon
- 2 tablespoons caramel
- Sugar free syrup ¼ tablespoon
- 2 tablespoons of almond flour
- 1 teaspoon of melted butter
- Pinch of salt and black pepper

HOW TO MAKE CREAMY CHEESE KETO WAFFLES?

- Take a blender, add 2 eggs
- Add 2 ounces of sour cream cheese in it
- Add ½ teaspoon of onion powder, cinnamon powder
- Add whipping cream, 2 tablespoons of caramel
- Add ¼ tablespoon of sugar free syrup
- Add 2 tablespoons of almond flour
- Add 1 teaspoon of melted butter
- Add a pinch of salt and black pepper in it
- Blend it until no lumps remain
- Heat up the Waffle maker and spray with almond oil
- Cook it for 5-6 minutes and then remove it pour maple syrup

6: NEXT LEVEL SWEET AND SPICY CHAFFLES?

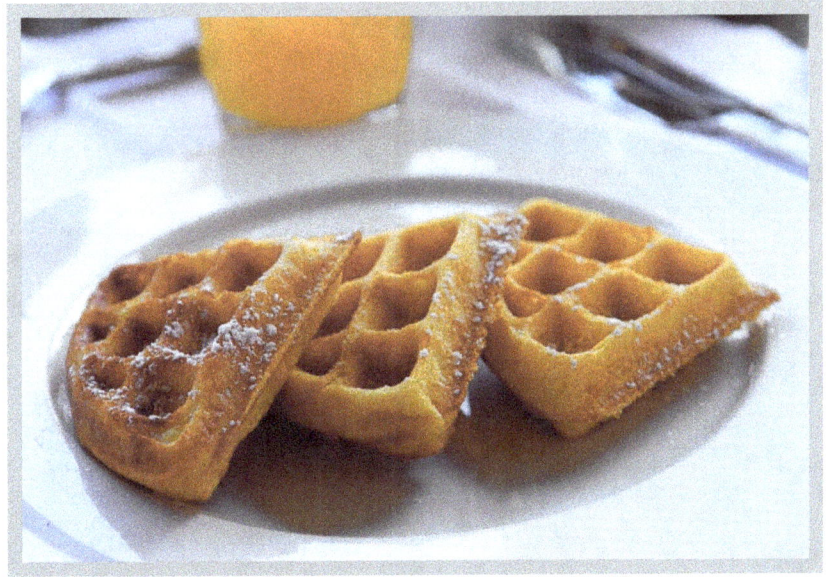

INGREDIENTS.

- 1 large egg
- ½ cup of Mozzarella cheese

- ½ teaspoon of psyllium husk powder
- ½ teaspoon unflavored protein
- ½ Quest cinnamon crunch protein
- 1 teaspoon vanilla extract
- ½ teaspoon baking powder
- 3 tablespoon almond flour
- 1 teaspoon of melted butter
- Pinch of salt and black pepper
- Honey 1 teaspoon

HOW TO MAKE NEXT LEVEL SWEET AND SPICY CHAFFLES?

- Take a blender and add 1 large egg
- Add ½ cup of Mozzarella cheese, ½ teaspoon of psyllium husk powder
- Add a teaspoon of unflavored protein
- Add ½ quest of cinnamon crunch protein
- Add 1 teaspoon of vanilla extract
- Add ½ teaspoon of baking powder
- Add 3 tablespoons of almond flour
- Add a pinch of salt and black pepper in it
- Blend it well until it gets mixed
- Heat up the Waffle maker and cook for 5-6 minutes
- Remove from the iron and pour some honey on it

7: BEST KETO CHAFFLES

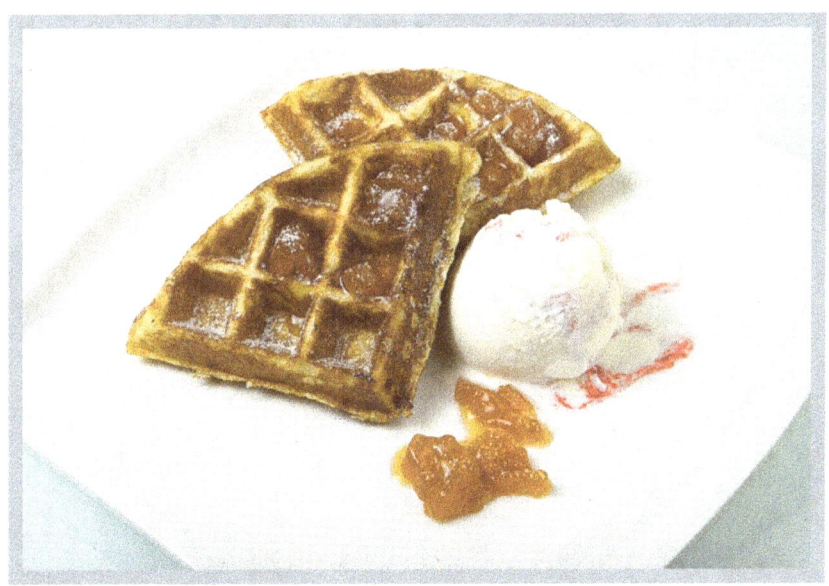

I**NGREDIENTS..**

- 2 eggs
- Heavy whipping cream ½ cup

- ½ cup Avocado oil
- ¼ teaspoon salt
- Coconut flour 2 tablespoons 15g
- Super-fine almond flour 224g
- Cream of tartar ¼ tablespoon
- Xanthan gum ¼ tablespoon
- Pure vanilla extract ¼ teaspoon
- ½ teaspoon baking soda
- Liquid staria 30 drops
- Sesame seeds 1 teaspoon

HOW TO MAKE BEST KETO CHAFFLES??

- Take a blender, add 2 eggs
- Add heavy whipping cream, avocado oil and ¼ teaspoon salt
- Add coconut flour, super-fine almond flour
- Add cream of tartar and Xanthan gum ¼ teaspoon
- Add pure vanilla extract
- Add ½ teaspoon baking soda
- Mix it well in blender until no lumps remain
- Heat up waffle maker and pour waffle batter sprinkle sesame seeds on it
- Cook it for 5-6 minutes then remove
- Pour liquid staria on it

8: CRISPY, CHEESEY AND SPICY CHAFFLES WITH A TOUCH OF SWEETNESS IN IT..

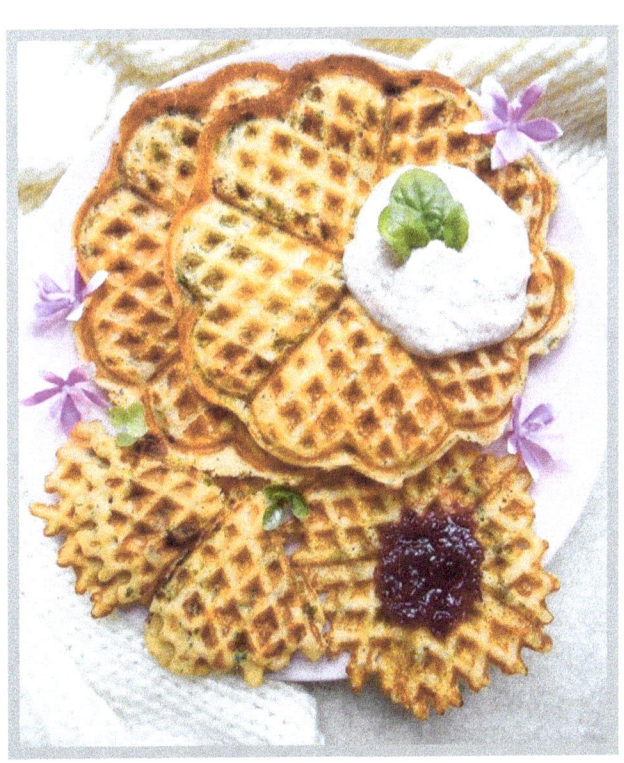

INGREDIENTS..

- 1 egg
- ½ cup Mozzarella cheese
- Cinnamon powder 1 teaspoon
- Nutmeg powder 1 teaspoon
- Ginger powder 1 teaspoon
- Vanilla extract ½ teaspoon
- Some garlic powder to give waffles the touch of garlic bread
- 1 tablespoon of crumbs of crispy bacon
- 1 tablespoon of chopped walnuts or pecans
- Butter cubes 2
- 1 teaspoon honey

HOW TO MAKE THESE CRISPY, CHEESEY AND SPICY CHAFFLES?

- Take a blender, add egg
- Then add Mozzarella cheese in it
- Add cinnamon powder, Nutmeg powder and vanilla extract in it
- Add garlic powder in it to give it the taste of garlic bread
- Add 1 tablespoon of walnuts and pecans in it
- Add honey in it
- Blend it until smooth mixture forms
- Heat up the waffle maker and pour waffle batter on it
- Sprinkle crumbs of crispy bacon on it
- Cook it for 4-5 minutes
- Remove from maker and top it with butter cubes

9: DELICIOUS KETO CHAFFLES..

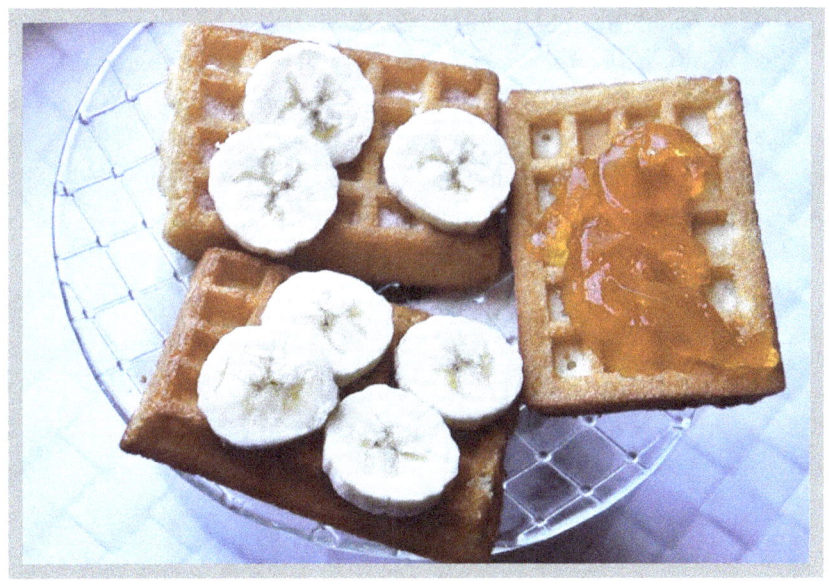

INGREDIENTS..

- 1 egg
- 1 tablespoon of melted but

- 1 tablespoon of coconut flour
- 1 tablespoon of almond flour
- 1 teaspoon of mustard powder
- ½ teaspoon of pork rind dust
- ½ teaspoon of caraway seeds
- 2 tablespoons of Mozzarella cheese
- ½ tablespoon of maple extract
- Tiny pinch pink salt as per taste

HOW TO MAKE DELICIOUS CHAFFLES??

- Take a bowl, add 1 egg, melted honey
- Add coconut flour, almond flour and mustard powder in it
- Add ½ teaspoon of pork rind dust
- Add ½ teaspoon of caraway seeds
- Add Mozzarella cheese in it
- Also add tiny pinch pink salt as per taste in it
- Whisk it well for 2 minutes until a smooth chaffle batter forms
- Take a waffle maker, spray some coconut oil
- Pour chaffle batter on it and cook it for 4-5 minutes
- Remove from maker and pour ½ tablespoon of maple extract on it

10: BLUE BERRIES CHAFFLE..

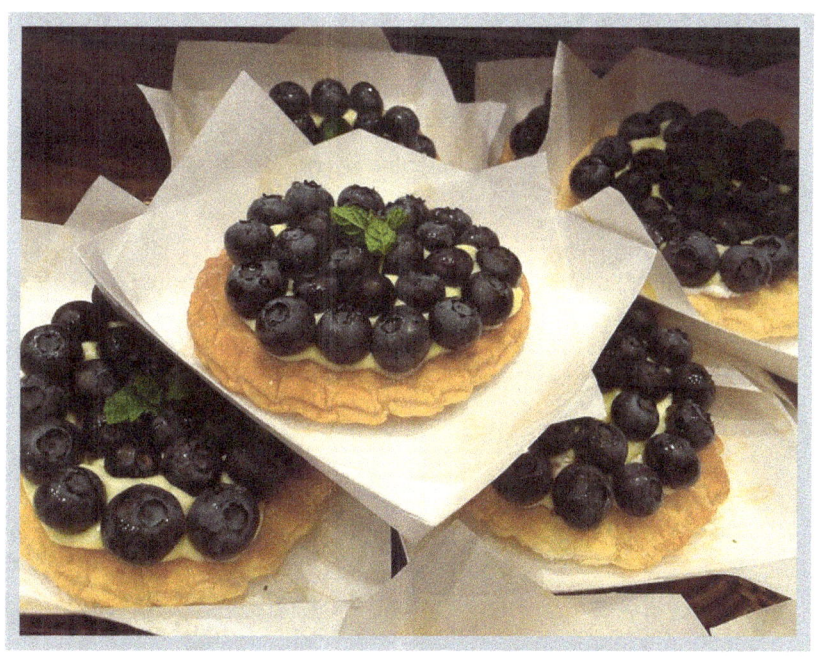

INGREDIENTS..

- 2 eggs
- Cream cheese softened
- 1 tablespoon sweetener
- 1 tablespoon coconut flour
- ¼ teaspoon of baking powder
- ¼ tablespoon of sweet dough extract
- ¼ teaspoon of organic blue berries powder
- Blue berries 4-4

HOW TO MAKE BLUE BERRIES CHAFFLE?

- Take a bowl, add 2 eggs
- Add Cream cheese softened
- Add 1 tablespoon of sweetener
- Add coconut flour, baking powder
- Also add ¼ tablespoon of sweet dough extract
- Add ¼ teaspoon of organic blue berries powder
- Mix it well
- Heat up waffle maker and pour a chaffle batter on it
- Put 4- 5 blue berries on it and cook it for 4-5 minutes

11: STANDARD CHAFFLE

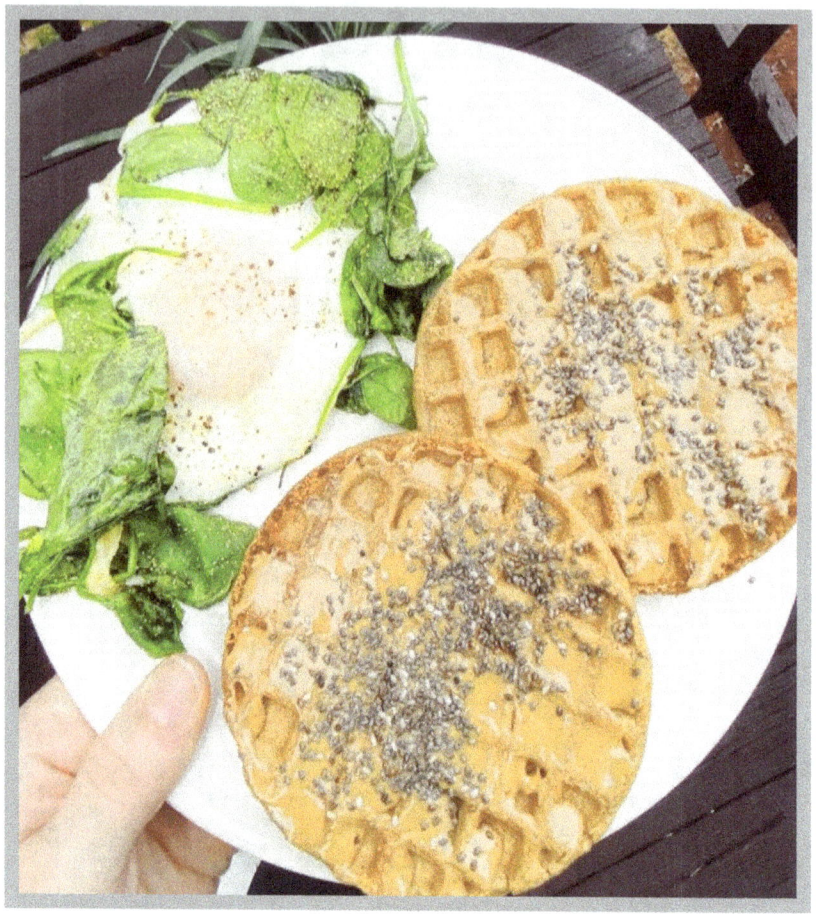

I**NGREDIENTS.**

- 1 egg
- Pinch of pink salt
- Coconut flour 2 tablespoons
- Honey ½ teaspoon
- Dry fruit mixture 1 tablespoon
- 1 teaspoon of melted butter
- Coconut oil ½ teaspoon

HOW TO MAKE STANDARD CHAFFLE?

- Take a blender, add 1 egg
- Add pinch of pink salt
- Add coconut flour
- Add honey in it
- Add dry fruit mixture in it
- Add 1 teaspoon of melted honey
- Blend it until smooth chaffle batter forms
- Heat up waffle batter and spray coconut flour on it
- Pour chaffle batter on it and cook it for 3-4 minutes

12: CHOCOLATE CHIP COOKIE CHAFFLES..

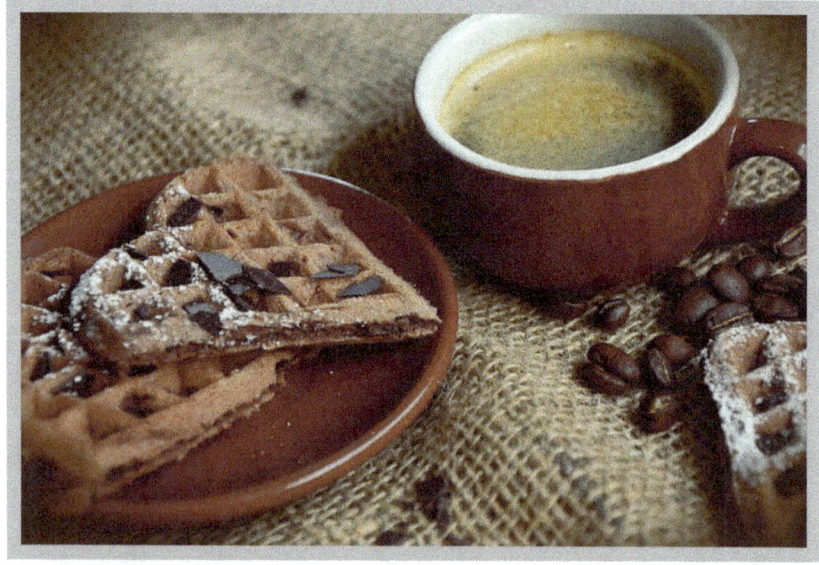

Ingredients..

- 1 egg
- ½ cup of shredded Mozzarella cheese

- 2 ½ teaspoon of brown sugar
- 1 teaspoon of vanilla extract
- 1 tablespoon of coconut flour
- 1 tablespoon of chocolate chips

HOW TO MAKE CHOCOLATE CHIP COOKIE CHAFFLES?

- Take a bowl, add 1 egg
- Add ½ cup of shredded Mozzarella cheese
- Add 2 ½ teaspoon of brown sugar in it
- Add vanilla extract
- Add 1 tablespoon of coconut flour in it
- Whisk it well until smooth batter forms
- Heat up waffle maker and sprinkle some coconut oil
- Pour chaffle batter and sprinkle chocolate chips on the batter
- Cook it for 4-5 minutes

13: BBQ KETO CHAFFLES

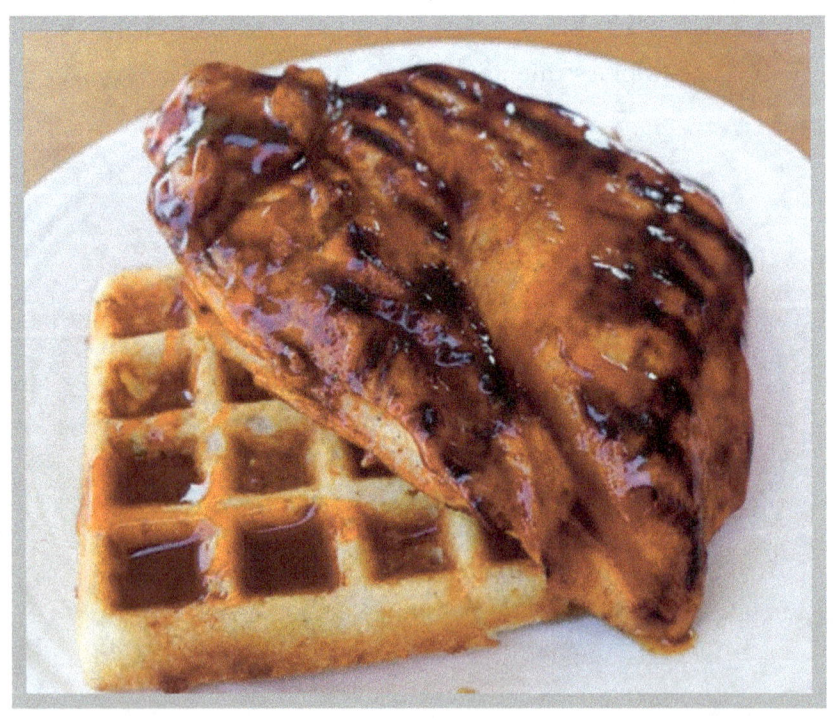

INGREDIENTS...

- 1 egg
- 1 cup of shredded Mozzarella cheese
- 1-2 tablespoons of Fish sauce / soy sauce
- ¼ cup of shredded chicken
- Pinch of salt
- Honey ½ teaspoon
- Black pepper ½ teaspoon
- 1 tablespoon almond flour

HOW TO MAKE BBQ KETO CHAFFLES?

- Take a bowl, add 1 egg
- Add 1 cup of shredded Mozzarella cheese
- Add fish sauce / Soy sauce
- Add ¼ cup of shredded chicken
- Add pinch of salt
- Add honey ½ teaspoon
- Add black pepper in it
- Add tablespoon almond flour
- Mix it well until it combines
- Heat up waffee maker and pour the Chaffle batter in it
- Cook it for 4-5 minutes

14: KETO CHICKEN BACON RANCH CHAFFLES..

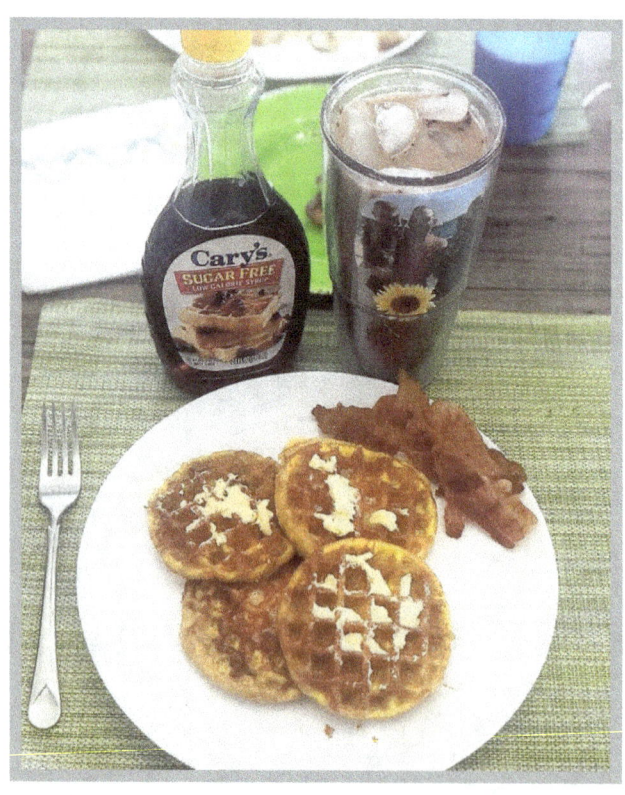

INGREDIENTS..

- 1 egg
- ½ cup of Mozzarella cheese
- 1-2 tablespoona of Ranch
- ¼ cup of Shredded chicken
- ¼ cup of bacon crumble's
- Honey ½ teaspoon
- Salt and black pepper 1 teaspoon
- Coconut powder 1 teaspoon

HOW TO MAKE KETO CHICKEN BACON RANCH CHAFFLE?

- Take a bowl, add 1 egg
- Add ½ cup of Mozzarella cheese
- Add 1-2 tablespoons of Ranch
- Add ¼ cup of Shredded chicken
- Add ¼ cup of bacon crumble's
- Add honey
- Add salt and black pepper in it
- At the end add coconut powder
- Mix all the ingredients well for 2-3 minutes
- Heat up waffle maker and spray some olive oil
- Pour chaffle batter and cook for 4-5 minutes

15: EASY KETO CHAFFEL RECIPE..

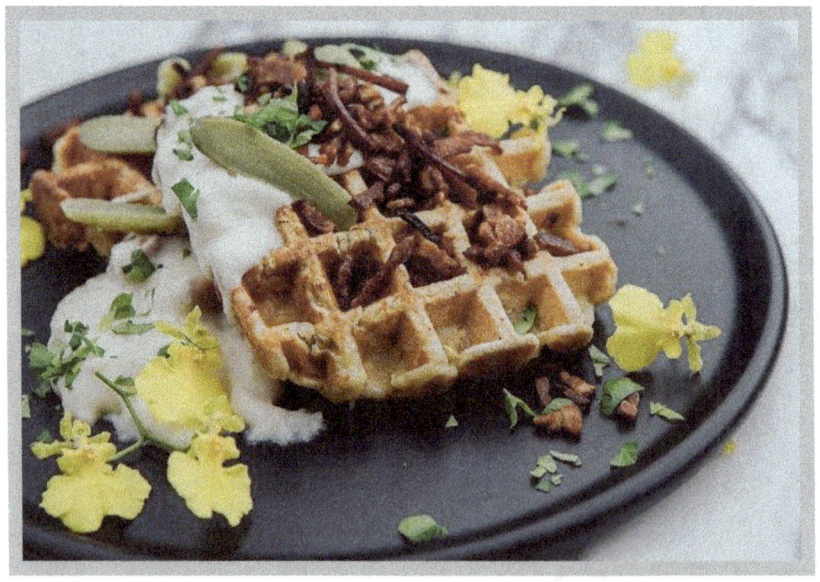

INGREDIENTS...

- 1 egg
- 1 cup Cheddar cheese

- ½ teaspoon garlic powder
- ½ seasoning powder
- 2 tablespoons coconut flour
- ¼ teaspoon baking powder
- Pinch of salt
- Thinly chopped peppers
- 1 teaspoon Keto friendly sweetener

HOW TO MAKE EASY CHAFFEL RECIPE?

- Take a bowl, broke one egg in it
- Add 1 cup of cheddar cheese
- Add garlic powder in it
- Add all seasoning powder
- Add coconut flour in it
- Add ¼ teaspoon baking soda
- Add a pinch of salt
- Whisk it well
- Heat up waffle maker, spray some coconut oil on it
- Pour the Keto chaffle batter and sprinkle some thinly chopped peppers on it
- Cook it for 4-5 minutes
- Pour some keto-friendly sweetener on it

16: KETO PIZZA STYLE CHAFFEL..

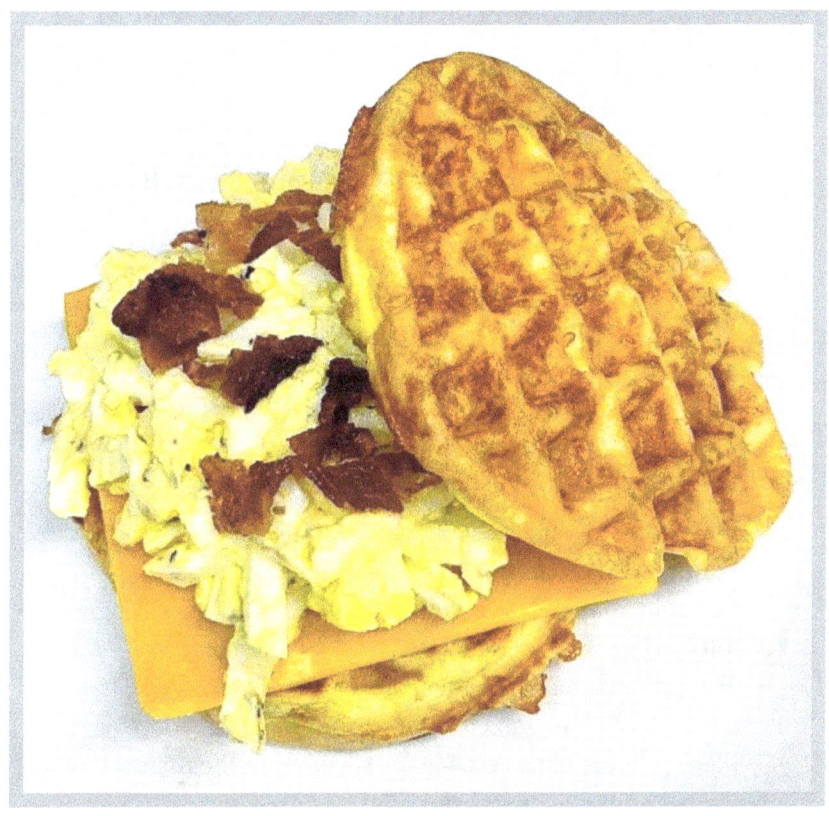

INGREDIENTS...

- 1 egg white
- 1 tablespoon coconut flour
- ½ cup Mozzarella cheese shredded
- 1 tablespoon cream cheese softened
- ¼ teaspoon baking powder
- ⅛ teaspoon seasoning powder
- ⅛ teaspoon garlic powder
- Pinch of salt
- 3 teaspoons Marina sauce
- ½ cup cheddar cheese
- 6 pepperonis cut in half
- 1 tablespoon Parmesan cheese shredded

- ¼ tablespoon basil seasoning
- ½ teaspoon coconut oil
- Tomato sauce ½ tablespoon

HOW TO MAKE KETO PIZZA STYLE CHAFFEL?

- Take a bowl, add egg white, coconut flour
- Add ½ cup of Mozzarella cheese in shredded form
- Add 1 tablespoon of cream cheese softened
- Add baking powder and pinch of salt
- Then after adding these ingredients mix them well
- Add Marina sauce, basil seasoning and cheddar cheese in it again mix them
- Heat up waffle maker, spray some coconut oil
- Pour the Chaffel batter and cook it for 3-4 minutes
- Carefully remove the Chaffel from the waffle maker, then follow the same instructions to make the second one
- Top each chaffel with tomato sauce, pepperoni, Mozzarella cheese and Parmesan cheese
- Place it in the oven on a baking sheet upon the top shelf of the oven for five or six min
- Following that step please turn the furnace to sear so that the cheese begins to bubble and brown
- Remove from the oven and sprinkle basil on top

17: BROCCOLI AND CHEDDAR LOW CARB KETO WAFFLES..

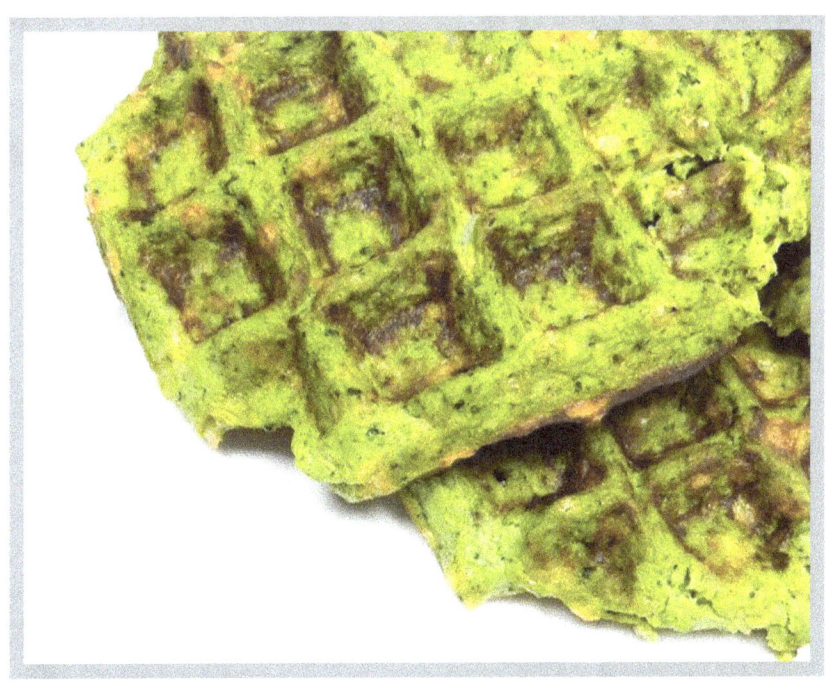

INGREDIENTS..

- 2 eggs, beaten
- ½ cup Mozzarella cheese shredded
- ½ cup triple cheddar cheese shredded
- 2 tablespoons Parmesan cheese, grated
- ½ teaspoon onion powder
- ½ cup broccoli, cooked and finely chopped
- 1 tablespoon Alfredo sauce
- ½ teaspoon salt and pepper
- 1 tablespoon cooked chicken (shredded)
- Creamy basil sauce ½ teaspoon

HOW TO MAKE BROCCOLI AND CHEDDAR LOW CARB KETO WAFFLES?

- Take a bowl add 2 beaten eggs
- Add Mozzarella cheese shredded
- Add triple chadder cheese shredded
- Add Parmesan cheese grated
- Add ½ teaspoon of onion powder
- Add cooked and finely chopped broccoli
- Add cooked chicken shredded
- Add pinch of salt and black pepper in it
- Mix all the ingredients well and add Alfredo sauce in it
- After mixing all the ingredients add creamy basil sauce also and mix it for 2 minutes
- Heat up waffle maker and sprinkle some triple cheddar cheese on it, then pour the chaffle batter and sprinkle some triple cheddar cheese
- Cook it for 5-6 minutes

18: LOW CARB KETO WAFFLES..

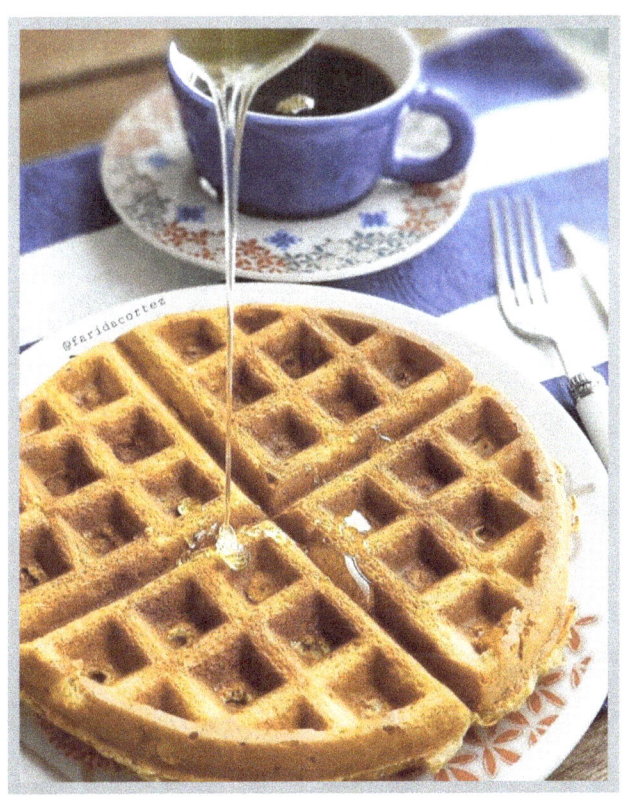

INGREDIENTS..

- 2 large eggs mixed
- 1 teaspoon of dried parsley
- ¼ teaspoon ground black pepper
- 56 g Mozzarella cheese shredded
- 56 g Cheddar cheese shredded

HOW TO MAKE LOW CARB KETO WAFFLES?

- Take a bowl, add 2 eggs mixed
- Add a teaspoon of dried parsley
- Add ¼ teaspoon of ground black pepper
- Add Mozzarella shredded cheese in it
- Add Cheddar cheese in it
- Mix all the ingredients well
- Heat the Waffle maker and spray some coconut oil
- Pour the batter and cook it for 5-6 minutes
- Serve with tomato slices and green onions

19: CAULIFLOWER WAFFLES..

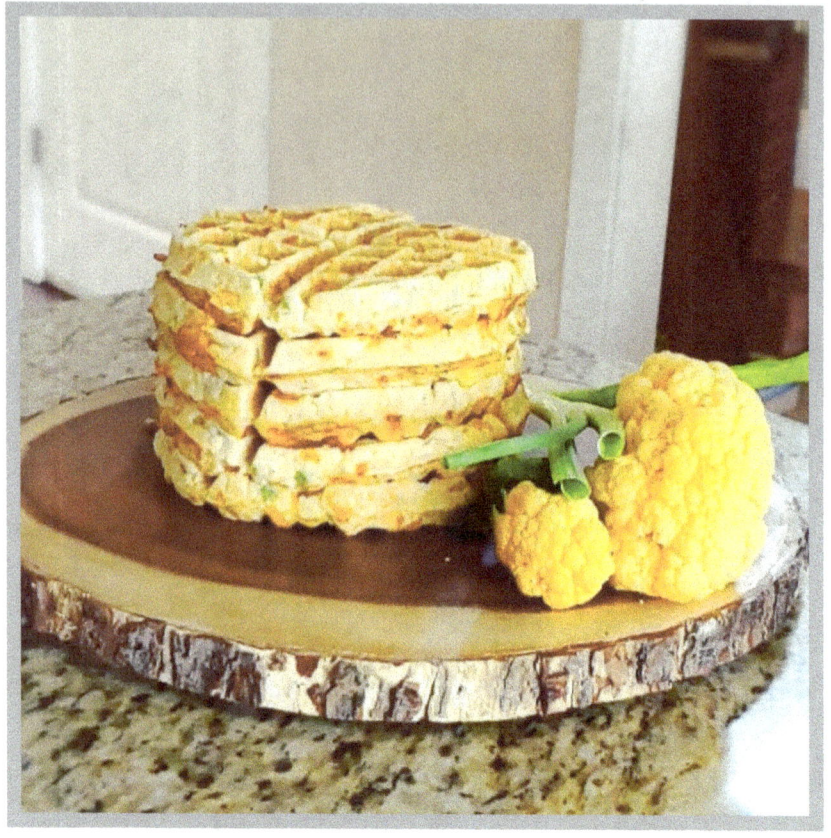

INGREDIENTS...

- 2 cups cauliflower grated
- 2 cups shredded Mozzarella cheese
- 2 eggs
- 2 tablespoons coconut flour
- ½ tablespoon of onion powder
- ½ teaspoon of ginger powder
- ½ teaspoon of oregano
- Pinch of salt and black pepper

HOW TO MAKE TASTY CAULIFLOWER WAFFLES?

- Cut the cauliflower in half and cut the florets from the other half
- Pulse the florets in a food processor until the cauliflower is minced and looks almost like rice
- Take a bowl add minced cauliflower
- Add 2 eggs, shredded Mozzarella cheese in it
- Add tablespoon of coconut flour
- Add ½ teaspoon of onion powder
- Add ½ teaspoon of ginger powder
- Add ½ teaspoon of oregano
- Add pinch of salt and black pepper in it
- Mix all the ingredients until well combined
- Heat up the Waffle maker and spray some coconut oil
- Pour the Waffle batter on it sprinkle some shredded Mozzarella cheese on it and cook for 5-6 minutes

20: SWEET POTATO WAFFLE'S..

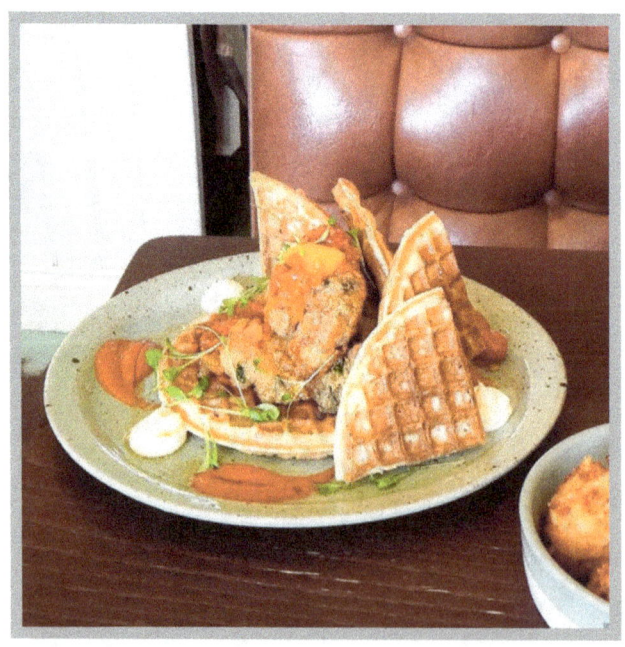

INGREDIENTS..

- 1 large sweet potato cooked (About ¾ of cup mashed)
- ½ cup of rolled oats
- ½ cup of coconut flour
- ½ cup of unsweetened almond milk
- 2 eggs
- 1 teaspoon of baking powder
- ¾ teaspoon of cinnamon powder
- ¼ teaspoon salt
- Cooking spray

HOW TO MAKE SWEET POTATO WAFFLES?

- Set waffle maker to preheat
- Combine cooked sweet potatoes and oats in a blender
- Blend until well combined
- Pour egg and milk into a blender with the sweet potatoes and oat base
- Blend until well combined, add the rest of ingredients and blend until fully poureed
- Spray waffle maker with cooking spray
- Pour the batter into waffle maker
- Cook for 4-7 minutes
- Let waffle cool on a baking rack
- Serve with whipped cream, maple syrup and pecans if desired

21: PUMPKIN SPICE KETO CHAFFLES..

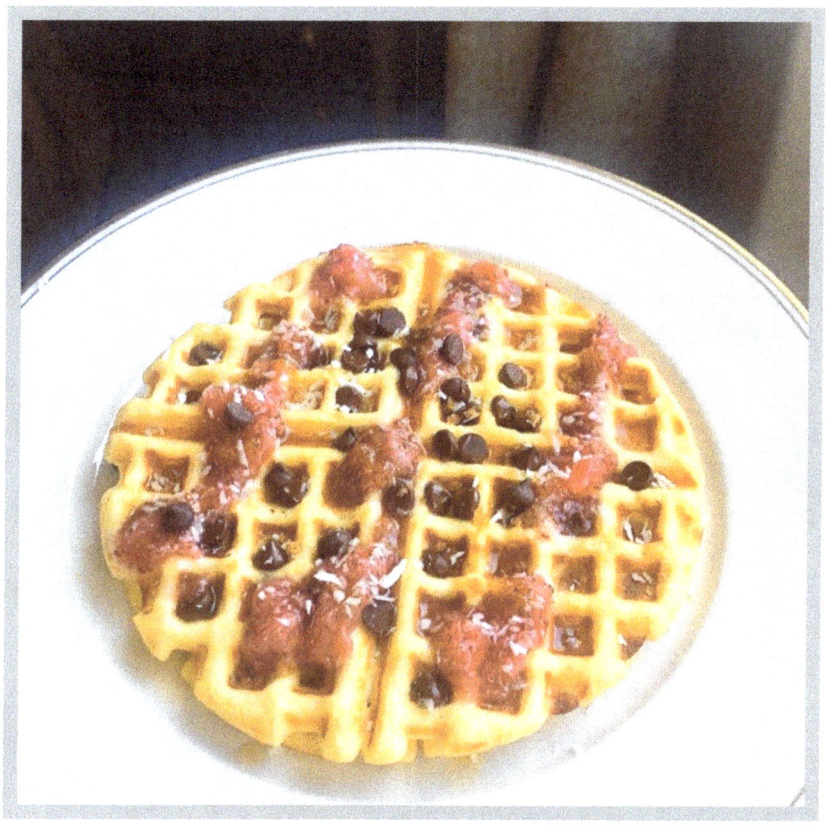

INGREDIENTS..

- 2 eggs
- 2 tablespoons pumpkin puree
- 1 tablespoon pumpkin spice
- 2 teaspoons coconut flour
- 1 teaspoon Vanilla extract
- 1 cup of finely shredded Mozzarella cheese
- Pinch of salt

HOW TO MAKE PUMPKIN KETO CHAFFLES..

- Take a bowl, add two eggs

- Give them a quick whisk
- Add 2 tablespoons of pumpkin puree
- Then add 1 tablespoon of pumpkin spice
- Add coconut flour and vanilla extract in it
- Add 1 cup of finely shredded Mozzarella cheese
- Add a pinch of salt
- Mix all the ingredients well combined
- Heat up the Waffle maker spray some coconut flour
- Pour the Waffle batter on it and cook it for 5-6 minutes

22: BACON, MUSHROOMS SMOKED CHAFFLES..

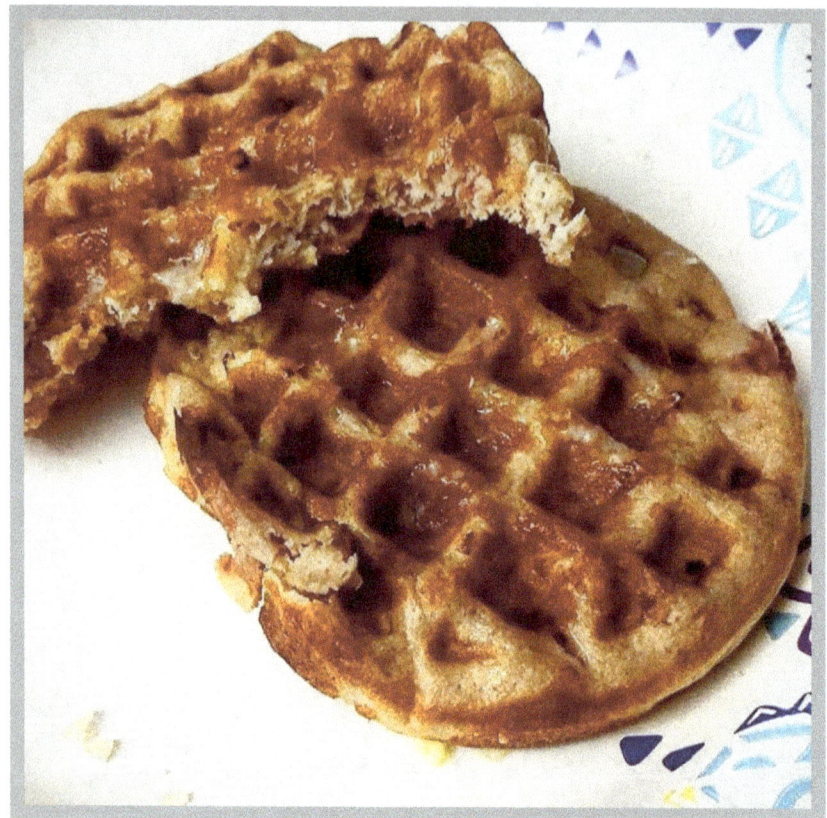

INGREDIENTS..

- 1 large egg
- ½ cup smoked shredded cheese
- 1 slice cooked bacon
- 2 tablespoons mushrooms diced
- 1 Green onion diced
- ½ teaspoon garlic powder
- Pinch of salt

HOW TO COOK BACON,MUSHROOMS SMOKED CHAFFLE?

- Take a food processor , add 1 large egg
- Add ½ cup smoked shredded cheese
- Add 1 chopped slice of cooked bacon
- Add 2 tablespoons of diced mushrooms
- Add chopped green onions
- Add ½ teaspoon of garlic bread
- Add a pinch of salt
- Blend it until well combined
- Heat up the Waffle maker and spray some coconut oil on it
- Pour the Waffle batter and cook it for 5-6 minutes

23: PECAN CINNAMON CHAFFEL WITH DELICIOUS CREAM CHEESE SOFTENING..

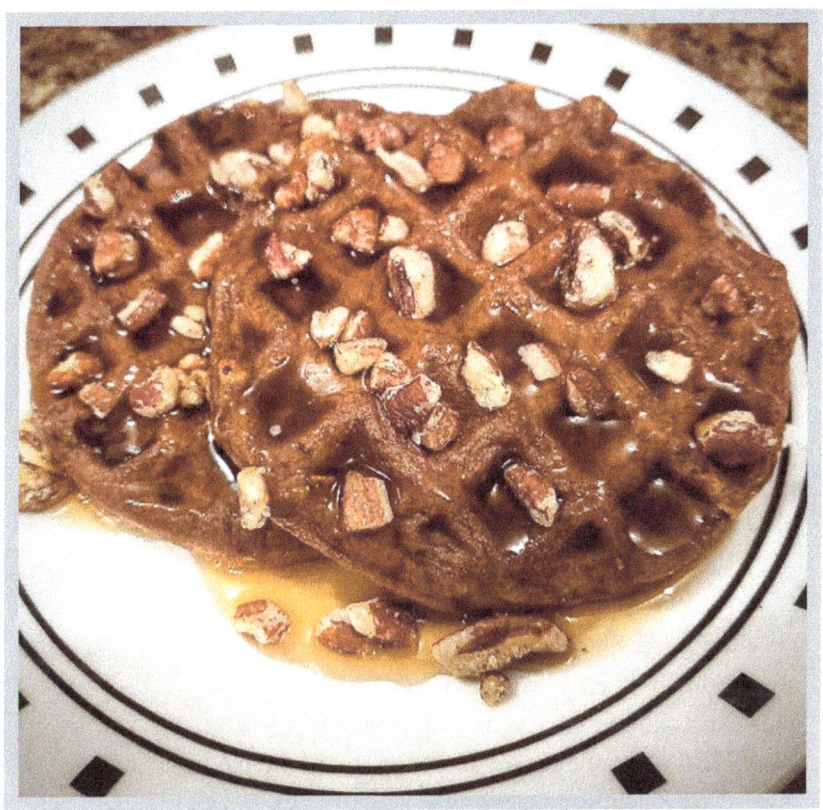

INGREDIENTS..

- 1 egg
- 1 tablespoon Almond flour
- 1 teaspoon coconut oil
- Pinch of salt
- 1 teaspoon of Vanilla extract
- 1 teaspoon heavy cream
- 1 teaspoon of Monk fruite powdered sweetener
- 1 teaspoon baking powder
- 1 teaspoon of cinnamon powder
- 5-6 pecans chopped

FROSTING..

- 1 ounce (2 teaspoon) Cream cheese softened
- 2 teaspoons butter softened
- 1 tablespoon heavy cream
- 1 teaspoon Monk fruite powdered sweetener
- Splash of vanilla extract
- ½ teaspoon of Maple syrup

HOW TO MAKE PECAN CINNAMON CHAFFEL WITH DELICIOUS CREAM CHEESE SOFTENING?

- Take a bowl, add egg
- Add almond flour then add coconut oil
- Add pinch of salt and vanilla extract
- Add heavy cream, 1 teaspoon of Monk fruite powdered sweetener
- Add 1 teaspoon of baking powder
- Add 1 teaspoon of cinnamon powder
- Add chopped pecans in it
- Mix all the ingredients with a beater
- Heat up waffle maker and pour the waffle batter then cook it for ⅚ minutes
- Till then prepare **FROSTING**
- Take a bowl add cream cheese and butter cubes in a microwave for a few seconds to melt them
- Add heavy cream and 1 teaspoon of Monk fruite powdered sweetener
- Splash some vanilla extract
- Then add maple syrup in it
- Mix all the ingredients well
- Remove the chaffles from the maker and pour the frosting on them

24: CHAFFEL PICKLE SPEARS..

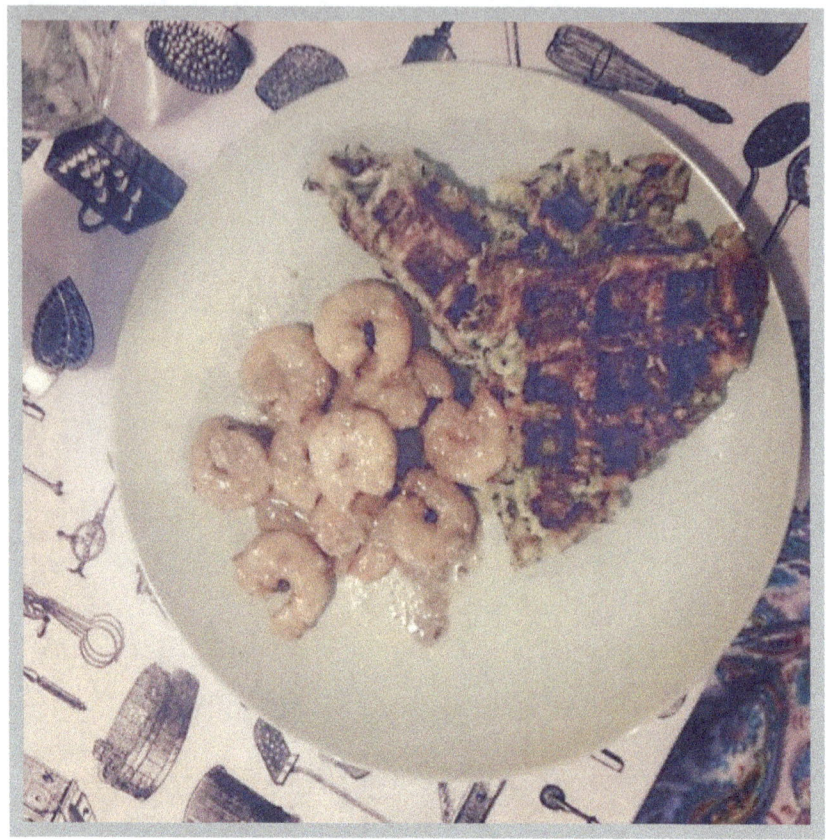

INGREDIENTS..

- 1 cup of coconut flour
- Pinch of salt
- 2 tablespoon's ground pork rinds
- 1 tablespoon of Monterey Jack Cheese
- 1 egg
- ½ teaspoon of Lemon juice
- 1 teaspoon of mustard powder
- ½ teaspoon of seasoning powder

HOW TO MAKE CHAFFEL PICKLE SPEARS?

- Take a bowl, add coconut flour
- Add 1 egg and pinch of salt
- Add mustard powder and seasoning powder
- Add lemon juice and ground pork rinds
- Add Monterey Jack Cheese
- Mix all the ingredients well until well combined
- Heat up the Waffle maker and spray some coconut oil
- Pour the waffle batter in the maker and cook it for 5-6 minutes

25: VEGETABLE CHEESE CHAFFLE.. INGREDIENTS...

- 2 egg
- 1 cup of almond flour
- 1 tablespoon of cooked pumpkin puree
- 2 tablespoons of Cheddar cheese
- 1 tablespoon of chopped onion
- 1 tablespoon of chopped capsicum
- ½ teaspoon garlic and ginger powder
- ½ tablespoon of chopped broccoli
- Pinch of salt and black pepper
- Lemon juice 1 tablespoon

HOW TO MAKE VEGETABLE CHEESE CHAFFLE?

- Take a bowl add one egg
- Add a cup of almond flour
- Add cooked pumpkin pure
- Add cheddar cheese, chopped onions
- Then add garlic and ginger powder in it
- Add chopped capsicum, chopped broccoli
- Add pinch of salt and black pepper
- Add some lemon juice
- Mic all the ingredients until well combined
- Heat up the Waffle maker

- Sprinkle some cheddar cheese then pour the batter again sprinkle some cheddar cheese on it
- Cook for 5-6 minutes

26: KETO GRILLED PEPPERONI CHAFFEL.. INGREDIENTS..

- 1 egg
- 1 cup of Mozzarella cheese
- 1 teaspoon of garlic powder
- 1 teaspoon of onion powder
- Pinch of salt and black pepper
- Fish sauce
- Few drops of honey
- 1 teaspoons of shredded chicken
- 5-6 slices of pepperoni

HOW TO MAKE KETO GRILLED PEPPERONI CHAFFEL?

- Take a bowl, add egg in it
- Add half cup of mozzarella cheese
- Then add onion and garlic powder
- Add pinch of salt and black pepper
- Add fish sauce, few drops of honey
- Add shredded chicken
- Mix them until well combined
- Heat up waffle maker and sprinkle some Mozzarella cheese then pour waffle batter on it again sprinkle Mozzarella cheese on it
- Cook it for 5-6 minutes
- Remove from the maker put pepperoni on it and again sprinkle some mozzarella cheese again put in the maker and cook for 2 minutes

27: KETO FRENCH TOAST LIKE CHAFFLES...

INGREDIENTS...

- 2 eggs
- Mozzarella cheese 1 cup
- Whipping cream 5 tablespoons
- Cinnamon powder 1 tablespoon
- Vanilla extract ½ teaspoon
- Sweetener 1 tablespoon
- Crushed dry fruits 1 tablespoon
- Coconut oil 1 teteteteaspoon

HOW TO MAKE FRENCH TOAST LIKE CHAFFLES?

- Take a bowl add eggs, dry fruits powder and mozzarella cheese and mix them
- Heat up chaffel maker and spray some coconut oil
- Pour the batter and cook for 5-6 minutes
- Remove the first chaffle
- Again pour the remaining chaffle batter and cook for 5-6 minutes
- Remove it and put it in a plate
- Take a bowl add whipping cream, cinnamon powder
- Also add vanilla extract sweetener
- Mix all the ingredients until well combined
- Now take a Piece of Chaffle and dip it in a mixture
- Put it in a preheated pan and cook for 3-4 minutes

28: CHOCOLATE PECAN CHAFFLE..
INGREDIENTS..

1. 2 eggs
2. ½ cup cheese
3. ¼ teaspoon baking powder
4. 2 tablespoons of almond flour
5. 1 teaspoon of cocoa
6. Splash of vanilla extract

7. 1 teaspoon Swere
8. 1 cube of butter, cream cheese
9. 1 tablespoon chopped pecans
10. 1 tablespoon of chocolate chips

HOW TO MAKE CHOCOLATE PECAN CHAFFLE?

- Take a bowl add eggs, cheese
- Add baking powder, almond flour
- Then add cocoa, splash of vanilla extract
- Add 1 teaspoon of Swere, 1 cube of butter, cream cheese
- Add chopped pecans in the same bowl
- Mix all the ingredients until well combined
- Heat up the Chaffel maker and pour the batter on it sprinkle some chocolate chips and cook for 5-6 minutes
- Remove from the maker and enjoy

29: ORANGE CINNAMON ROLL CHAFFLE..
INGREDIENTS..

- 1 egg
- 1 tablespoon of almond flour
- ¼ teaspoon baking powder
- 1 teaspoon of psyllium husk powder
- 1 teaspoon of Orange extract
- ½ cup Mozzarella cheese
- ¼ teaspoon orange zest
- Chia seeds, hemp seed per taste

FROSTING..

- 5 teaspoons cream cheese
- Sugar powder 1 teaspoon
- ½ teaspoon orange extract
- Orange zest ¼ teteaspoon

HOW TO MAKE ORANGE CINNAMON ROLL CHAFFLE?

- Take a bowl, add egg, 1 tablespoon of almond flour
- Add baking powder, psyllium husk powder
- Add orange extract, ¼ teaspoon of orange zest
- Mix all the ingredients until well combined
- Heat up the Chaffle maker and pour this Chaffle batter
- Sprinkle Chia seeds and hemp seed
- Cook for 5-6 minutes
- Now prepare **FROSTING**
- Take a bowl, add cheese cream
- Sugar powder
- Add orange extract and orange zest
- Mix then well
- Remove the Chaffle from the maker and pour the **FROSTING** on it

25: VEGETABLE CHEESE CHAFFLE..

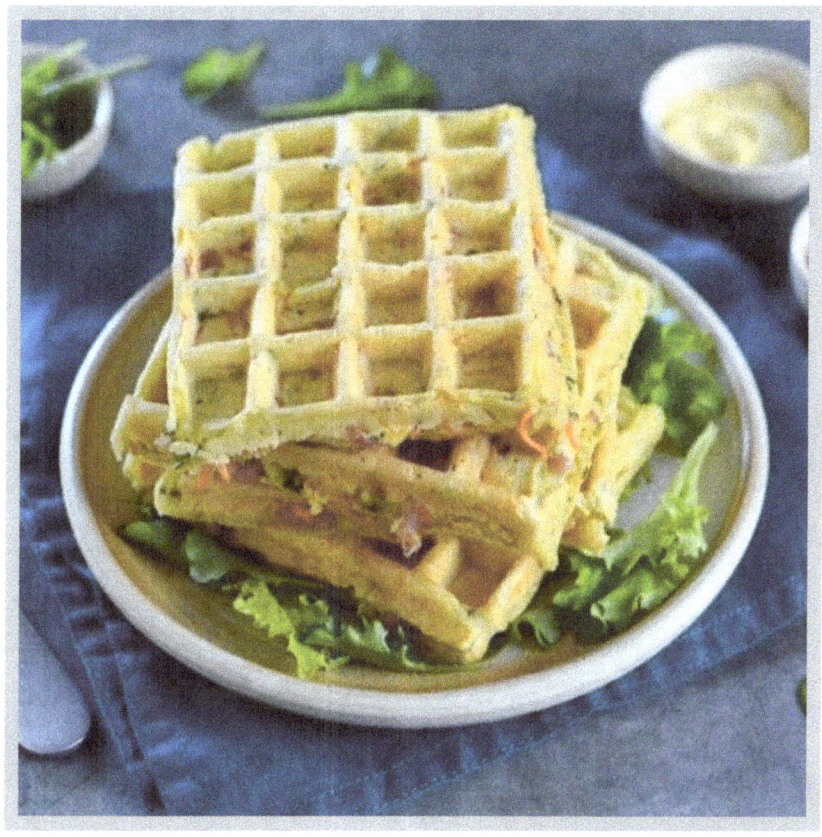

INGREDIENTS...

- 2 egg
- 1 cup of almond flour
- 1 tablespoon of cooked pumpkin puree
- 2 tablespoons of Cheddar cheese
- 1 tablespoon of chopped onion
- 1 tablespoon of chopped capsicum
- ½ teaspoon garlic and ginger powder
- ½ tablespoon of chopped broccoli
- Pinch of salt and black pepper
- Lemon juice 1 tablespoon

HOW TO MAKE VEGETABLE CHEESE CHAFFLE?

- Take a bowl add one egg
- Add a cup of almond flour
- Add cooked pumpkin pure
- Add cheddar cheese, chopped onions
- Then add garlic and ginger powder in it
- Add chopped capsicum, chopped broccoli
- Add pinch of salt and black pepper
- Add some lemon juice
- Mic all the ingredients until well combined
- Heat up the Waffle maker
- Sprinkle some cheddar cheese then pour the batter again sprinkle some cheddar cheese on it
- Cook for 5-6 minutes

26: KETO GRILLED PEPPERONI CHAFFEL..

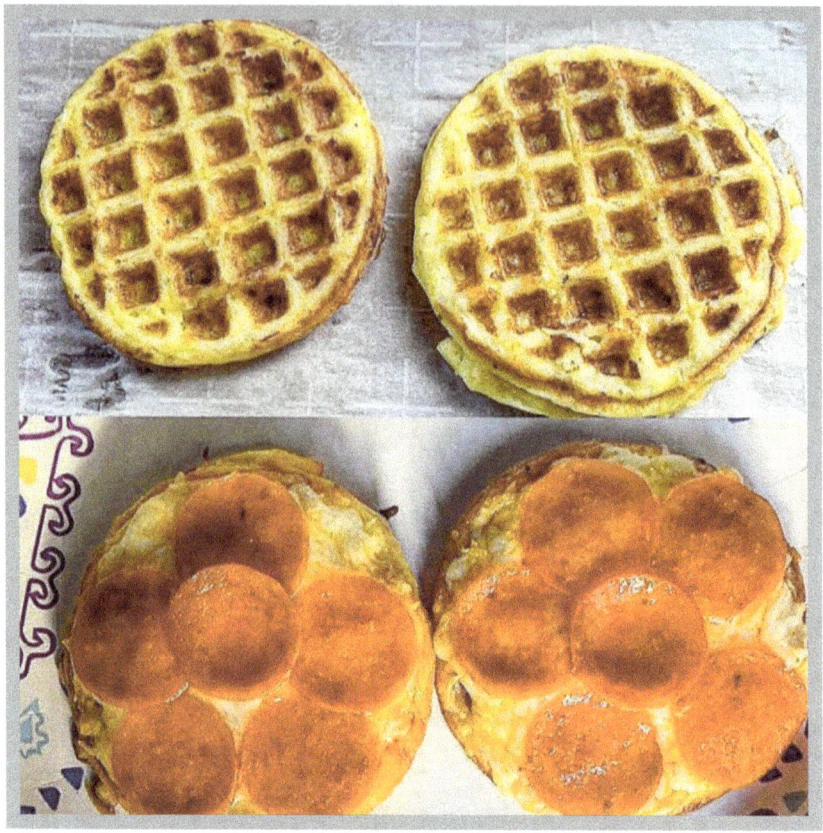

INGREDIENTS..

- 1 egg
- 1 cup of Mozzarella cheese
- 1 teaspoon of garlic powder
- 1 teaspoon of onion powder
- Pinch of salt and black pepper
- Fish sauce
- Few drops of honey
- 1 teaspoons of shredded chicken
- 5-6 slices of pepperoni

HOW TO MAKE KETO GRILLED PEPPERONI CHAFFEL?

- Take a bowl, add egg in it
- Add half cup of mozzarella cheese
- Then add onion and garlic powder
- Add pinch of salt and black pepper
- Add fish sauce, few drops of honey
- Add shredded chicken
- Mix them until well combined
- Heat up waffle maker and sprinkle some Mozzarella cheese then pour waffle batter on it again sprinkle Mozzarella cheese on it
- Cook it for 5-6 minutes
- Remove from the maker put pepperoni on it and again sprinkle some mozzarella cheese again put in the maker and cook for 2 minutes

27: KETO FRENCH TOAST LIKE CHAFFLES...

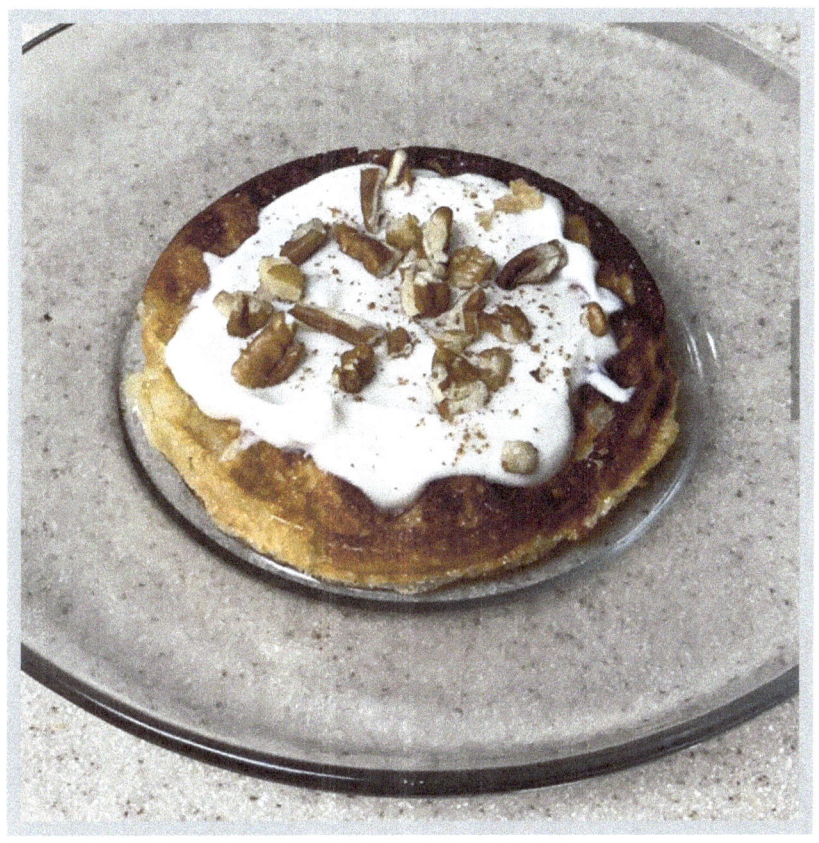

INGREDIENTS...

- 2 eggs
- Mozzarella cheese 1 cup
- Whipping cream 5 tablespoons
- Cinnamon powder 1 tablespoon
- Vanilla extract ½ teaspoon
- Sweetener 1 tablespoon
- Crushed dry fruits 1 tablespoon
- Coconut oil 1 teteteteaspoon

HOW TO MAKE FRENCH TOAST LIKE CHAFFLES?

- Take a bowl add eggs, dry fruits powder and mozzarella cheese and mix them
- Heat up chaffel maker and spray some coconut oil
- Pour the batter and cook for 5-6 minutes
- Remove the first chaffle
- Again pour the remaining chaffle batter and cook for 5-6 minutes
- Remove it and put it in a plate
- Take a bowl add whipping cream, cinnamon powder
- Also add vanilla extract sweetener
- Mix all the ingredients until well combined
- Now take a Piece of Chaffle and dip it in a mixture
- Put it in a preheated pan and cook for 3-4 minutes

28: CHOCOLATE PECAN CHAFFLE..

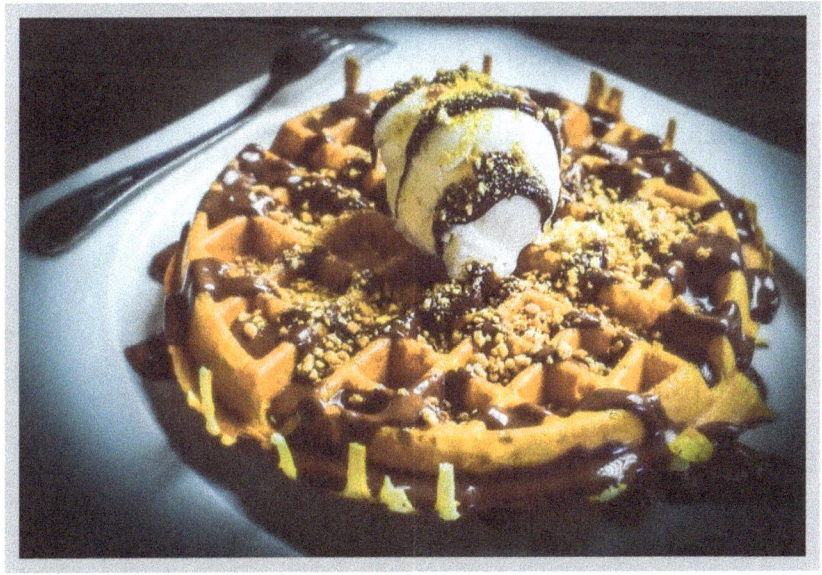

Ingredients..

1. 2 eggs
2. ½ cup cheese

3. ¼ teaspoon baking powder
4. 2 tablespoons of almond flour
5. 1 teaspoon of cocoa
6. Splash of vanilla extract
7. 1 teaspoon Swere
8. 1 cube of butter, cream cheese
9. 1 tablespoon chopped pecans
10. 1 tablespoon of chocolate chips

HOW TO MAKE CHOCOLATE PECAN CHAFFLE?

- Take a bowl add eggs, cheese
- Add baking powder, almond flour
- Then add cocoa, splash of vanilla extract
- Add 1 teaspoon of Swere, 1 cube of butter, cream cheese
- Add chopped pecans in the same bowl
- Mix all the ingredients until well combined
- Heat up the Chaffel maker and pour the batter on it sprinkle some chocolate chips and cook for 5-6 minutes
- Remove from the maker and enjoy

29: ORANGE CINNAMON ROLL CHAFFLE..

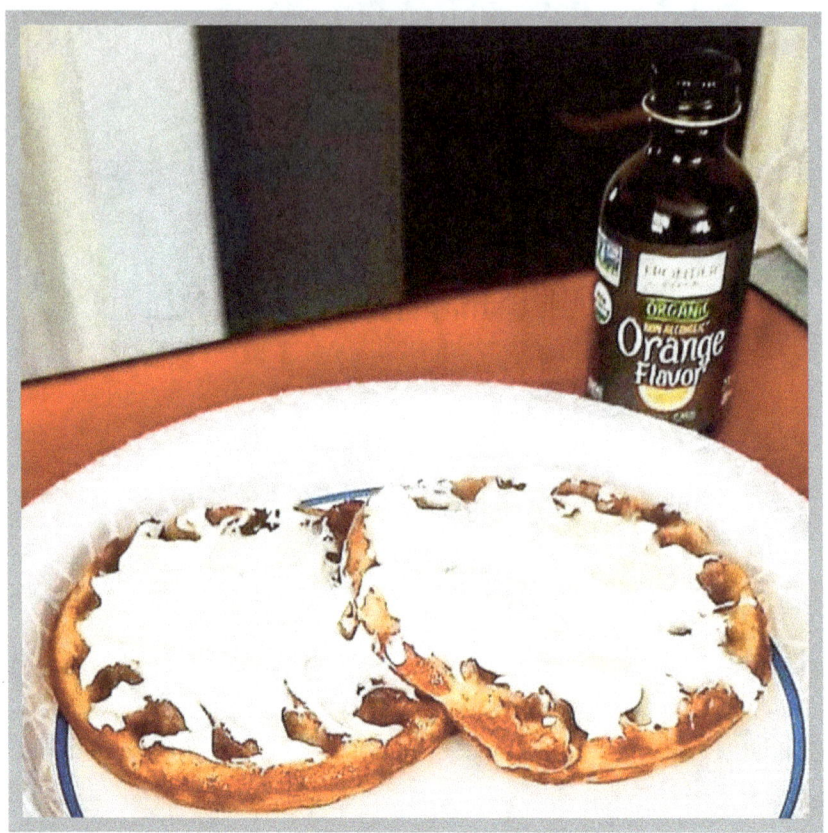

INGREDIENTS..

- 1 egg
- 1 tablespoon of almond flour
- ¼ teaspoon baking powder
- 1 teaspoon of psyllium husk powder
- 1 teaspoon of Orange extract
- ½ cup Mozzarella cheese
- ¼ teaspoon orange zest
- Chia seeds, hemp seed per taste

FROSTING..

- 5 teaspoons cream cheese
- Sugar powder 1 teaspoon
- ½ teaspoon orange extract
- Orange zest ¼ teteaspoon

HOW TO MAKE ORANGE CINNAMON ROLL CHAFFLE?

- Take a bowl, add egg, 1 tablespoon of almond flour
- Add baking powder, psyllium husk powder
- Add orange extract, ¼ teaspoon of orange zest
- Mix all the ingredients until well combined
- Heat up the Chaffle maker and pour this Chaffle batter
- Sprinkle Chia seeds and hemp seed
- Cook for 5-6 minutes
- Now prepare **FROSTING**
- Take a bowl, add cheese cream
- Sugar powder
- Add orange extract and orange zest
- Mix then well
- Remove the Chaffle from the maker and pour the **FROSTING** on it

30: KETO CORN BREAD CHAFFLE..

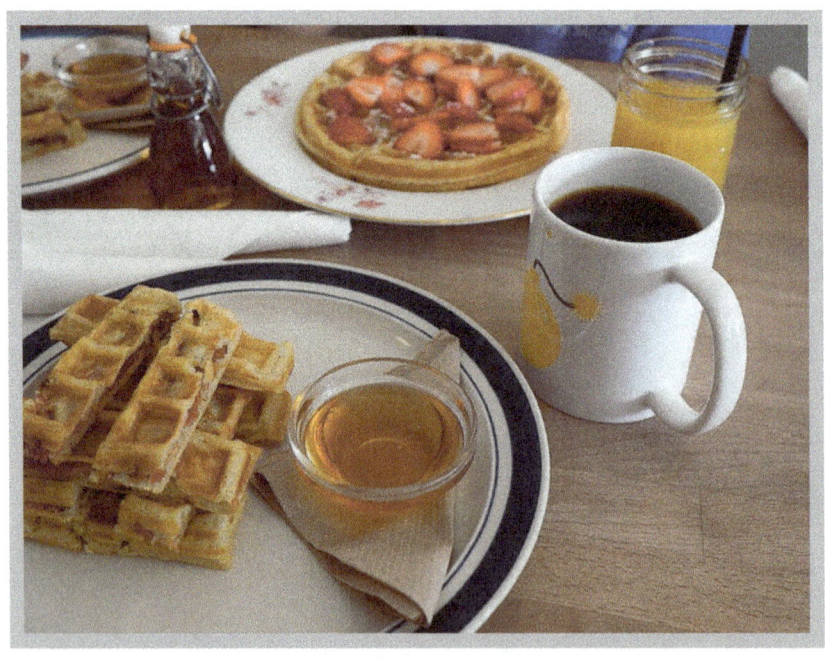

INGREDIENTS..

- 1 egg
- ½ cup cheddar cheese shredded
- ¼ teaspoon baking powder
- ¼ teaspoon cinnamon powder
- ¼ teaspoon corn bread extract
- Pinch of salt and black pepper
- Coconut powder ½ teaspoon

HOW TO MAKE KETO CORN BREAD CHAFFLES?

- Take a bowl, add egg
- Add cheddar cheese shredded
- Add baking powder, cinnamon powder
- Then add pinch of salt and black pepper
- Add coconut powder
- Add corn bread extract
- Mix all the ingredients until well combined
- Heat up the chaffle maker, pour the chaffle batter sprinkle some cheese and cook it for 5-6 minutes

www.ingramcontent.com/pod-product-compliance
Lightning Source LLC
Chambersburg PA
CBHW072208100526
44589CB00015B/2424